All About
MANAGING TYPE 2 DIABETES

By Laura Flynn R.N., B.N., M.B.A., in consultation with her nurse educator associates and physicians who assisted in contributing and editing.

ISBN No: 978 1 896616 60 5

© 2011 Mediscript Communications Inc.

The publisher, Mediscript Communications Inc., acknowledges the financial support of the Government of Canada through the Canadian Book Fund for our publishing activities.

Printed in Canada

www.mediscript.net

Book and Front Cover design by:
Brian Adamson, www.AdamsonGraphics.net

ALL ABOUT BOOKS
Trusted • Reliable • Certified

- 40+ titles available
- Comply with accreditation and regulatory bodies
- Suitable for caregivers, boomers with elderly parents, health workers, auxiliary health staff & patients
- Self study style with "test yourself" section
- Health On the Net (HON) certified

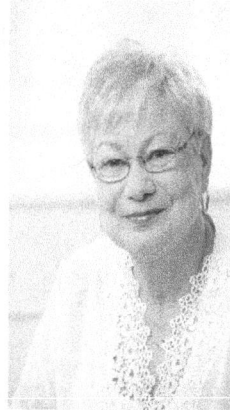

Some of our titles:

Alzheimers Disease	Arthritis	Multiple Sclerosis
Pain	Strokes	Elder Abuse
Falls Prevention	Incontinence	Nutrition & Aging
Personal Care	Positioning	Confusion
Transferring people	Care of the Back	Skin Care

For complete list of titles go to www.mediscript.net

Contact: 1 800 773 5088
Fax 1800 639 3186 • Email; mediscript30@yahoo.ca

CONTENTS

CORE CONTENT

INTRODUCTION

This book provides basic, non controversial and trusted information that can help a wide spectrum of readers.

The primary objective of the information is to help a person provide effective quality care to a loved one or someone in his or her care.

After reading this material you will have greater confidence in your caregiving role and will know what to do to help a person with Type 2 diabetes manage this health condition.

All the information is reliable and was written by a group of eminent nurse educators who ensured the information complies with best practice guidelines and satisfies the various accreditation and regulatory bodies. Because there is so much unreliable information on the internet, you can be assured the "All About" publications are HON (Health On the Net) certified.

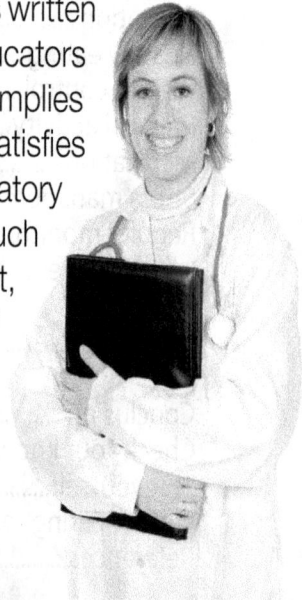

This book can be an invaluable aid to:

- A caregiver caring for a relative or friend;
- A health worker seeking a reference aid;
- A patient or person with Type 2 diabetes;
- Any person involved in health care wishing to expand his or her knowledge.

SOMETHING TO THINK ABOUT...

The secret of life isn't what happens
to you, but what you DO with what
happens to you.

Dr. Norman Vincent Peale

AN IMPORTANT MESSAGE
FROM THE PUBLISHER

Each person's treatment, advice, medical aids, physical therapy and other approaches to health care are unique and highly dependant upon the diagnosis and overall assessment by the medical team.

We emphasize therefore that the information within this book is not a substitute for the advice and treatment from a health care professional.

This book provides generic information concerning the issues around Type 2 diabetes and common sense, well-established care practices for people with this condition.

With all this in mind, the publishers and authors disclaim any responsibility for any adverse effects resulting directly or indirectly from the suggestions contained within this book or from any misunderstanding of the content on the part of the reader.

HAVE YOU HEARD

The following words don't exist, but we think they should:

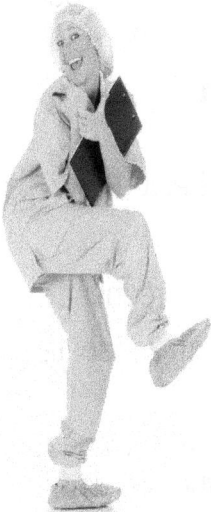

- AQUADEXTROUS (ak wa deks 'trus) adj. Possessing the ability to turn the bathtub tap on and off with your toes.

- DISCONFECT (dis kon fekt') v. To sterilize the piece of candy you dropped on the floor by blowing on it, assuming this will somehow 'remove' all the germs.

- FRUST (frust) n. The small line of debris that refuses to be swept onto the dust pan and keeps backing a person across the room until he finally decides to give up and sweep it under the rug.

- TELECRASTINATION (tel e kras tin ay' shun) n. The act of always letting the phone ring at least twice before you pick it up, even when you're only 6 inches away.

HOW MUCH DO YOU KNOW?

It helps to figure out how much you know before you start. In this way you will have an idea as to the gaps in your knowledge prior to reading the content. Please circle to indicate the best answer. Remember, at this stage, you are not expected to know all the answers:

1. What is the best definition of "Type 2 diabetes"?

a. A viral disease

b. A type of diabetes that occurs during pregnancy

c. A type of diabetes that stems from a genetic disorder

d. A condition in which the body either cannot produce insulin or cannot use the insulin it produces

2. Which statement about Type 2 diabetes is most true?

a. It is treated with pills only.

b. It is no longer a serious disease.

c. The incidence of Type 2 diabetes is on the decline.

d. It is becoming more common among young people.

3. What is the best definition of ``nephropathy``?

a. Disease of the eye

b. Kidney disease

c. Nerve disease

d. Poor circulation

4. What is the most common form of diabetes?

a. Type 1 diabetes

b. Type 2 diabetes

c. Gestational diabetes

d. All forms of diabetes occur at the same rate

5. Which of the following is a risk factor for Type 2 diabetes?

a. Obesity

b. Smoking

c. Viral infection

d. Diet low in calcium

6. Disease of the large blood vessels can cause which diabetic complication over time?

a. Coronary artery disease

b. Retinopathy

c. Nephropathy

d. Neuropathy

7. Which statement about hypoglycemia is most true?

a. It refers to high blood glucose.

b. Symptoms appear slowly.

c. It occurs from not taking enough insulin.

d. It requires immediate attention.

ANSWERS

1. d. Diabetes is all about insulin which affects how much sugar is in your blood.

2. d. This is an alarming statistic and probably related to lifestyle.

3. b. Nephropathy is the technical name for kidney problems.

4. b. Also called adult onset diabetes, Type 2 diabetes is the most common by far.

5. a. Obesity, especially around the belly, seems to be a major risk factor for Type 2 diabetes.

6. a. The heart has many large blood vessels at risk from the complications of diabetes.

7. d. Hypoglycemia can be an emergency because people can faint or pass out due to very low blood sugar levels.

WHEN SOMEONE HAS TYPE 2 DIABETES

Diabetes mellitus is a chronic disorder that causes hyperglycemia (high blood sugar). Sugar (glucose) is the fuel that gives cells energy. Insulin is a hormone that assists the cells in the body to use sugar. Insulin helps keep the glucose level in the blood within normal levels. Hyperglycemia develops when the body is unable to produce or use insulin properly.

In persons with diabetes, glucose builds up in the blood instead of entering the cells. The cells become starved for energy, and the high blood glucose levels can cause serious problems over time.

The three main types of diabetes are Type 1, Type 2 and gestational diabetes.

Type 1 diabetes

With Type 1 diabetes, the body is unable to produce insulin. This type of diabetes can happen at any age although it usually affects children or young adults.

Type 2 diabetes

Type 2 diabetes occurs when the body cannot produce enough insulin or, alternately, cannot use the insulin that is produced.

Gestational diabetes

This type of diabetes develops during pregnancy and usually resolves after the baby is born.

Sometimes diabetes stems from surgery, drugs, malnutrition, genetic conditions or various other illnesses. About 1% to 5% of all diagnosed cases can be traced to these sources.

SOME WORDS TO KNOW

Acanthosis nigricans – a skin disease marked by darkened patches of skin, common in the neck, groin and armpit

Cerebrovascular disease (CVD) – a disease affecting the blood supply to the brain

Coronary artery disease (CAD) – an abnormal condition that affects the heart's arteries

Hyperglycemia – high blood sugar

Hypoglycemia – low blood sugar

Insulin resistance – a condition in which the pancreas produces insulin but the body cannot use it

Nephropathy - disease of the kidneys

Neuropathy - nerve damage

Pancreas – a gland that secretes substances, including insulin

Peripheral vascular disease (PVD) – a condition that results in poor circulation especially in the lower legs and feet

Polycystic ovary syndrome – a hormonal condition that can cause infertility and other health problems in women

Postprandial – after a meal

Retinopathy - an eye disease that can lead to a loss of vision

Schizophrenia – a chronic mental disorder that can result in disorganized thoughts and behavior

ABOUT TYPE 2 DIABETES

Type 2 diabetes usually starts with "insulin resistance". The pancreas produces insulin but the body cannot use it. The cause of insulin resistance is not known. Because the body cannot use insulin to bring sugar into the cells, the level of sugar within the blood rises. In response to an increase of sugar in the blood, the pancreas produces extra insulin that the body still cannot use. Over time, the cells that produce insulin in the pancreas (beta cells) wear out. Insulin production slows down and causes insulin deficiency.

Type 2 diabetes used to be called "adult-onset diabetes" because the condition was generally diagnosed over the age of forty. However, it is becoming more common among young adults and even adolescents. In the past 10-15 years the prevalence of Type 2 diabetes in children has increased at least ten-fold in the United States. It is increasing in Canada as well, particularly among Aboriginal youth. It now affects as many as 1% of Canadian Aboriginals between 5 and 18 years of age.

Non-insulin dependent diabetes mellitus (NIDDM) is another term that was often used to describe Type 2 diabetes. The term is no longer used as many clients with Type 2 diabetes do require insulin injections to regulate their condition.

14.6 million people in the U.S. have been diagnosed with diabetes. It is estimated that about another 6.2 million have the disease but have not yet been diagnosed. Over 2 million people in Canada have the disease. Type 2 diabetes, the most common form of this disease, accounts for 90-95% of all the diagnosed cases of diabetes. Because Type 2 diabetes develops slowly over time, many people do not notice any symptoms for a number of years.

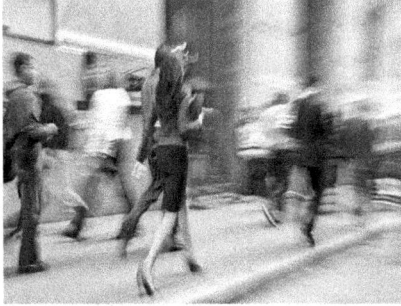

The rapid rise of Type 2 diabetes is cause for concern. The prevalence of this type of diabetes has increased by 49% over the past decade. This change has been linked to the increase in overweight and obesity in the population.

RISK FACTORS

There is no known cause for Type 2 diabetes. It occurs more often in persons over the age of forty and is also more common among certain ethnic groups. In the U.S., persons of Hispanic, Native American, African American, Asian American, or Pacific Islander descent are particularly at risk. High risk groups in Canada include persons of Aboriginal, Hispanic, Asian, South Asian, or African descent.

Other risk factors include:

- High blood pressure (140/90 mm Hg or higher)
- Family history (first-degree relative such as a parent or sibling)
- Obesity (especially excess fat around the waist)
- History of gestational diabetes or having had a child with a birth rate of over 9 lbs. (4 kg.)
- History of impaired glucose tolerance or impaired fasting plasma glucose (These are blood tests that measure blood glucose levels)
- Certain abnormal lipid (fat) levels

The Canadian Diabetes Association lists several other factors that increase the risk of Type 2 diabetes. These are a previous diagnosis of:

- Polycystic ovary syndrome
- Acanthosis nigricans (darkened patches of skin)
- Schizophrenia

CONSIDER FOR A MOMENT . . .

What risk factors are present

in your own life?

PREVENTION

Many persons have blood glucose levels that are higher than usual although not high enough to be diagnosed with diabetes. This condition is called "pre-diabetes". Pre-diabetes often leads to Type 2 diabetes over time.

Persons with pre-diabetes are at risk of developing heart disease and death. 50% already have disease of the heart and major blood vessels by the time they are diagnosed with diabetes. Another 25% develop it later on. So early detection of Type 2 diabetes is very important. Persons 65 years and over are advised to have their blood glucose level tested on an annual basis.

A person at risk of developing Type 2 diabetes can take steps to prevent it. Lifestyle changes can lower blood glucose levels in pre-diabetes and positively affect some of the other factors present in metabolic syndrome.

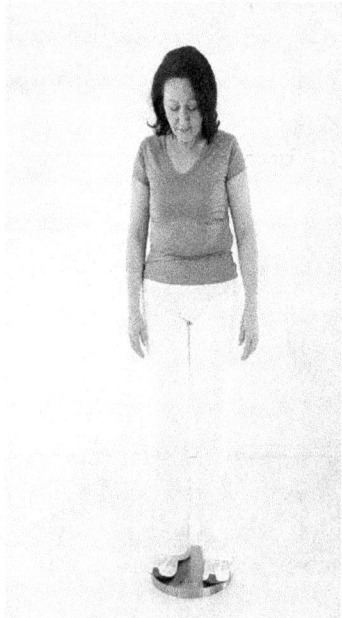

Full-blown diabetes does not have to occur.

Having extra weight, especially around the waist, is one of the risk factors for Type 2 diabetes. About 90% of patients who develop Type 2 diabetes are obese. The main reason for overweight and obesity is consuming too many calories and following an inactive lifestyle.

Research has shown that lifestyle changes that focus on diet and exercise can prevent or delay the onset of Type 2 diabetes. Some studies revealed a 58% decrease of Type 2 diabetes among those who made positive lifestyle changes.

CONSIDER FOR A MOMENT . . .

What lifestyle changes could you
make to promote your health?

SYMPTOMS

Signs of Type 2 diabetes usually appear slowly. These symptoms develop due to high levels of sugar in the blood and include:

- Thirst
- Increased urination
- Hungry
- Feeling tired
- Blurred vision
- Pain, tingling, burning, and loss of sensation
- Cuts and sores that are slow to heal
- Weight loss

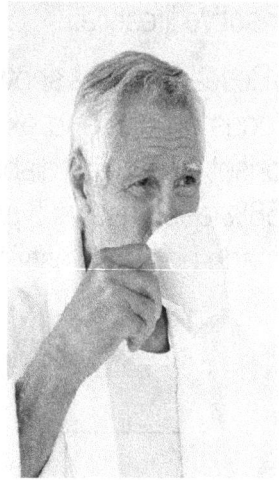

Some people with Type 2 diabetes have no symptoms at all. They discover they have the disease following routine blood work or only after they have developed complications, such as blurred vision or heart problems.

COMPLICATIONS

Uncontrolled diabetes may lead to many complications over time. People with diabetes are now living longer so complications are becoming more common. Complications from diabetes arise from damage to the large blood vessels as well as damage to the small blood vessels.

Complications arising from damage to large blood vessels include:

Coronary artery disease (CAD)

CAD can lead to heart attack which is often silent in persons with diabetes. The person could have a heart attack without any symptoms at all. In the absence of usual symptoms such as pain and shortness of breath, the person may not seek medical attention. The death rate from heart disease is two to four times higher for persons with diabetes.

Cerebrovascular disease (CVD)

CVD could lead to stroke, which tends to be more severe in persons with diabetes. Stroke can cause paralysis to one side of the body, difficulty with speech and understanding. Diabetes greatly increases the risk of stroke.

Peripheral vascular disease (PVD)

PVD results in poor circulation especially in the lower legs and feet. The decreased circulation can lead to poor healing. Foot ulcers often occur and are slow to heal. Some clients develop complications that lead to amputation over time.

Complications from small vessel damage include:

Retinopathy

Retinopathy is an eye disease that can lead to a loss of vision. In many cases, diabetic retinopathy is already present by the time the person is diagnosed with Type 2 diabetes. Diabetic retinopathy accounts for 12,000 to 24,000 new cases of blindness in the U.S. each year.

Nephropathy

Nephropathy refers to disease of the kidneys. 20-40% of persons with diabetes eventually develop nephropathy. Kidney disease due to diabetes sometimes develops into kidney failure. This means that the kidneys can no longer function on their own and the patient would require a kidney transplant or dialysis.

Neuropathy

Neuropathy refers to nerve damage. Nerve damage can result in loss of feeling, tingling, pain, and numbness, especially in the feet and lower legs. Damage can occur to some of the body organs such as the bladder and stomach. Nerve damage can also cause impotence.

Also:

73% of persons with diabetes have high blood pressure. Many suffer from gum disease. With uncontrolled diabetes, infections are more common and more difficult to treat. Cuts and sores heal more slowly.

HYPERGLYCEMIA AND HYPOGLYCEMIA

Uncontrolled diabetes can lead to episodes of hyperglycemia and hypoglycemia. Hyperglycemia refers to high blood sugar. Hypoglycemia refers to low blood sugar, sometimes called "insulin reaction". Both conditions can be very serious. You need to know the signs of both and notify a health care professional if you notice that someone in your care has these symptoms.

Hyperglycemia

Often occurs as the result of an infection or not taking enough insulin. Symptoms include thirst, frequent urination and fatigue. Symptoms appear slowly. Hyperglycemia is usually not an emergency situation. In the absence of treatment, however, it can progress and it can lead to coma and possibly death. The blood sugar level should be checked and treatment started as soon as possible. Treatment may include the administration of insulin.

Hypoglycemia

Hypoglycemia may occur from taking too much insulin or oral diabetic agent, taking the drug at the wrong time, not eating enough or eating at the wrong times. Symptoms of hypoglycemia often develop suddenly and include:

- Fast pulse
- Pounding heartbeat
- Anxiety
- Shakiness
- Sweating
- Tingling sensations (in the mouth or extremities)
- Headache
- Nausea
- Hunger
- Weakness

There may be difficulty with concentrating and reasoning, slurring of speech, blurred vision, dizziness and sleepiness. A severe hypoglycemic reaction can result in loss of consciousness and seizures.

What to do

This is an emergency situation and needs to be treated right away. Treatment for mild to moderate hypoglycemia consists of giving 15 grams of glucose (or carbohydrate that contains glucose) to an adult. Table 1 outlines several examples of 15 grams of carbohydrate. Giving any of these products will raise a person's blood sugar level. The values cited in the Clinical Practice Guidelines for Canada (2003) differ slightly from those found in the U.S. sources. For that reason, the table outlines both recommendations.

Table 1 – Examples of 15 grams of carbohydrate

US	CANADA
2-3 glucose tablets	15 g of glucose in the form of glucose tablets
1/2 cup of fruit juice	175 ml. (3/4 cup) of juice
1/2 cup of soda (regular, not diet)	3/4 cup of regular soft drink (regular, not diet)
1 cup of skim milk	
1-2 tsps. of sugar or honey	15 ml. (3 teaspoons) or 3 packets of table sugar dissolved in water 15 ml. (1 tablespoon) of honey
a packet or tube of glucose gel	
5-6 pieces of hard candy	6 Life Savers (1=2.5 g of carbohydrate)

The blood glucose should be checked again 15 minutes after giving the carbohydrate. If still low, another 15 grams of carbohydrate should be given. The person should eat a meal within an hour.

If the person becomes unconscious:

- Do not inject insulin or give food or fluids by mouth.

- Inject 1 mg. of glucagon to raise blood sugar if you have been instructed how and when to do so.

- Get the help of a professional. The person may need extra supervision, even possibly hospital admission, for awhile. You may have to monitor his blood glucose level for some time.

If your family member is living in a health care facility, check out the policies and procedures for treating hyperglycemia and hypoglycemia.

DAILY CARE

Once the diagnosis of diabetes is made, a plan to manage the diabetes is needed. Managing diabetes requires a team effort that may involve professionals such as the physician, diabetic educator, nutritionist, pharmacist, ophthalmologist, nurse practitioner, endocrinologist, etc. Type 2 diabetes is often described as a self-managed disease. That means that your family member is a very important person in the management of the disease and will often be involved in glucose monitoring, medications, diet, exercise, and care of the feet.

The person with diabetes, her family members and you, the caregiver, should consider the following:

✓ Know what diabetes is

✓ Know what the management care plan is

✓ Be able to recognise the symptoms that would require emergency care

✓ Know who to contact in an emergency. The telephone numbers for these people should be easily accessible.

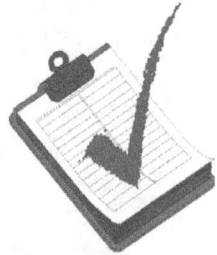

You will need to follow the plan of care and, if your family member is living in a health care facility, you will need to follow the policies and procedures of that facility as well.

As a caregiver, you can help by encouraging and supporting your family member to follow the management plan. Participating in keeping daily records of blood sugar levels, food intake and activities is also important. Many people at home or in long term care facilities are confused, feeble, or ill so that you and other team members may need to assume greater responsibility for maintaining this person's health.

EDUCATION

Living a healthy lifestyle is very important. The person with Type 2 diabetes needs to be educated about making healthy choices. Information should include what symptoms to watch for, healthy eating, weight control, exercise needs, regular monitoring, medications, and general care needs. This information is available from various organizations, such as your local diabetes association. With information, your family member can be more involved in managing her care. Family, friends, and caregivers should also know general information about Type 2 diabetes. Your loved one should carry medical identification at all times.

CONSIDER FOR A MOMENT . . .

Where can you go to get information about diabetes?

HEALTHY EATING

Healthy eating can go a long way towards controlling diabetes. The focus should be on controlling glucose levels, losing any excess weight, limiting the intake of saturated fats, and eating healthy foods. Most people will benefit from increasing their consumption of whole grain products and vegetables, using unsaturated oils and choosing water over juices and soft drinks. Encourage your loved one to eat healthy foods and to cut back on fat, salt, and sugar. Paying attention to portion size is also important.

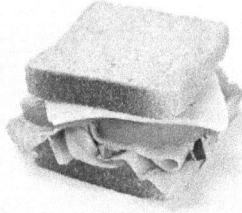

Ideally, a registered dietitian should assess the person's diet on an annual basis. The meal plan should be flexible and must be suited to his taste. People with Type 2 diabetes don't have to give up all their favorite foods but they will have to eat them in moderation. You may be asked to help keep a record of foods eaten over a certain period of time.

If your family member lives at home, you may be involved in preparing healthy and tasty meals. The American Diabetes Association (www.diabetes.org) has nutrition information and recipes on their website.

WEIGHT CONTROL

A healthy weight is another important factor in the control of diabetes. A balance must be kept between food, exercise, and medication. When a person is overweight, more insulin is needed to maintain blood sugar to the cells. Excess weight, especially around the waist, is also one of the risk factors of Type 2 diabetes.

People who are overweight should get advice from a health professional. Even a minor weight loss (5-10%) can improve blood glucose levels. A loss of weight may allow the person with Type 2 diabetes to avoid the need to take medication. You can encourage weight control and can help monitor your family member's weight.

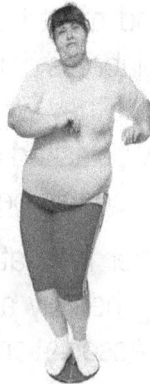

PHYSICAL ACTIVITY

Regular physical activity is helpful because it increases the production of insulin. Exercise also controls body weight, reduces blood sugar, lowers blood pressure, and reduces stress.

Encourage the person to choose a physical activity that is enjoyable. An enjoyable exercise will help to keep him interested in doing it. Gardening, swimming, dancing, and even doing household chores increase activity levels and have positive health benefits. Walking is a popular choice among older adults and has many added benefits:

- It can be done at the person's own pace
- It doesn't cost any money
- It can be done indoors (e.g. shopping mall) or outside

Due to chronic health concerns, many older people will be restricted in the amount of physical activity that they can do. In cases like these, chair-based exercises may be the best option.

An added bonus of exercise is that it helps the person's mental as well as physical health. Encourage your family member to check with her doctor prior to beginning a new exercise regime.

MEDICATIONS

For some people, diet and exercise alone may not produce the desired results. Medication may be helpful in those cases.

Many persons with Type 2 diabetes take oral medication to help control blood glucose levels. Insulin injections are used when oral agents, regular physical activity, and nutrition do not provide adequate control. Some people are able to achieve desired blood glucose levels through diet and exercise alone.

STRESS MANAGEMENT

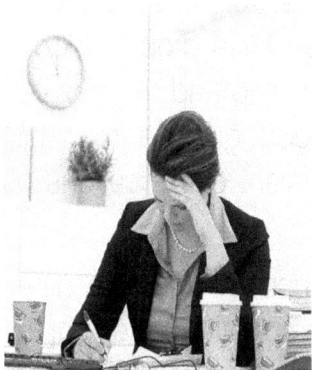

Stress can cause blood sugar levels to rise in persons with Type 2 diabetes. Stress also causes blood pressure to rise and has other negative health effects. Exercise and activities can reduce stress. The diabetic person should become involved in activities and programs to reduce stress. Some activities to reduce stress include walking, yoga, meditating, relaxing, or participating in an enjoyable hobby.

Help the person to keep a positive attitude. Be pleasant, supportive, and positive. She will need lots of support, especially when first diagnosed with the disease. Listen to her and encourage her involvement in activities that help to reduce stress. Some people find it helpful to take a few deep breaths when under stress. Others listen to music or take a relaxing bath. There are also health clinics and supportive groups that can offer helpful advice to persons with diabetes.

REGULAR MONITORING

A glucose monitor is used to test blood sugar levels. The tip of the finger is pricked for a drop of blood. The blood is applied to a test strip and the monitor reads the strip. Keeping blood glucose readings within normal levels helps prevent complications of diabetes.

Recommended blood glucose values differ depending on the time the person ate. For example, the desired range will be lower before eating and higher within two hours of ingesting a meal. Table 2 below gives the recommended plasma glucose target values for most people. It is important to note that these goals may not apply to everyone. The person's physician may set goals that differ in individual cases. It is also important to note that these "target values" do change from time to time based on new research findings.

Table 2 – Target values for plasma glucose levels

	US	CANADA
Fasting	90-130 mg/dl	4.0-7.0 mmol/L
Postprandial (after a meal)	<180 mg/dl	5.0-10.0 mmol/L

Your family member may be taught how to do glucose monitoring at home. You may be required to do the test if the he is unable to do it. You may also participate in keeping good records of the times and results of the tests.

The physician may also want to monitor blood pressure, cholesterol, and blood lipids on a regular basis. Another common blood test is an AIC which shows the level of glucose control over the past 2-3 months. Improved control in all of these areas can lower the risk of heart disease, stroke and other conditions. Persons with diabetes should see their physician on a regular basis. They should also have regular eye checkups.

INFECTION PREVENTION AND SKIN CARE

High blood sugar levels lower the ability of the white blood cells to fight off infections. Due to poor circulation in the blood vessels, the skin heals slowly. Nerve damage reduces feeling, which causes numbness. The person with Type 2 diabetes may not be able to sense if water is too hot, if shoes are too tight, or that he/she has been hurt. Special attention must be given to preventing injuries and to healing infections as soon as they are noticed. Ensure the environment is as safe as possible to avoid possible injury.

Good skin care, especially of the leg and the foot, is necessary to prevent and care for infections. Leg ulcers develop easily due to poor supply of blood to that area. If sores develop, they may not heal, which could lead to gangrene and possible amputation. Therefore, foot care is very important. Carefully inspect the feet and lower legs every day. Report any sore or injury right away. The diabetic person may require foot care by a health professional. Shoes should be worn at all times and they should fit well to avoid putting pressure on any part.

CASE EXAMPLE

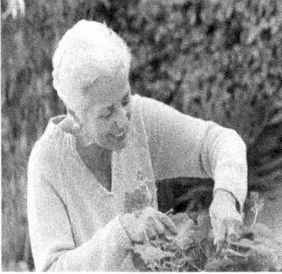

Sarah Johnson is 77 years old and lives at home. She receives insulin for Type 2 diabetes. She monitors her glucose levels and keeps a record to show her doctor at regular visits. According to these records, she has had a couple of episodes of hypoglycemia (low blood sugar). You have been asked to visit regularly and assist with management of her condition. On your first visit with her, you notice that Mrs. Johnson's appetite is poor and she has very little food in her house.

Why do you think Mrs. Johnson may be having episodes of low blood sugar?

What are some things that you, as a caregiver, can do to help her manage her condition?

YOUR ANSWERS TO CASE EXAMPLE

SUGGESTED ANSWERS TO CASE EXAMPLE

Why do you think Mrs. Johnson may be having episodes of low blood sugar?

Hypoglycemia (low blood sugar) may occur from one or all of the following:

• Taking too much insulin or oral diabetic agent

• Taking medication at the wrong time

• Not eating enough

• Eating at the wrong times

In Mrs. Johnson's case, her episodes of low blood sugar may be caused by the fact that she is eating poorly.

What are some things that you, as a caregiver, can do to help her manage her condition?

• Encourage her to follow the meal plan outlined by her nutritionist.

• Find out why she is not eating well. You may be able to suggest ways to resolve the problem. For example, if her appetite is poor because she dislikes eating alone, maybe she can share some meals with family or friends.

- Consider whether or not she needs help with shopping. Perhaps a family member or friend may be able to assist her with this task.

- Many communities have non profit agencies that offer a meal delivery program. Through this program, hot meals are delivered to seniors for a fee. Find out if there is a program in the area and if Mrs. Johnson would like to use it.

- Assist her to check blood glucose levels as instructed.

- Assist her to keep an accurate record of blood glucose readings.

- Find out if she knows the symptoms of low blood sugar and what to do if her blood sugar is low. If not, review them with her. Ensure she keeps a list of the symptoms and follow-up instructions in a prominent place.

- Find out what her plan of care states and reinforce it.

CONCLUSION

Once known as an "adult-onset" disease, Type 2 diabetes is now becoming much more common among younger persons. The increase in overweight and obesity is contributing to the rapid growth in the number of persons affected by Type 2 diabetes. Positive lifestyle changes can serve to prevent or delay the onset of the disease.

Uncontrolled diabetes can lead to many complications that are often difficult to treat. Managing diabetes requires a team effort that may involve many professionals. Type 2 diabetes is often described as a self-managed disease. That means that the person with diabetes is a very important person in the management of the disease.

CONSIDER FOR A MOMENT . . .

Take a few minutes and think about what

you have learned from this book.

Try to think of at least two things

that will help you with

your family member.

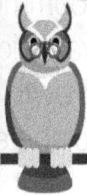

CHECK YOUR KNOWLEDGE

1. Define Type 2 diabetes.

2. Identify three risk factors for Type 2 diabetes.

3. Describe three possible complications from diabetes.

4. What are the signs of hyperglycemia and hypoglycemia?

5. Discuss three important aspects of daily care.

TEST YOURSELF

Please circle to indicate the best answer:

1. Which statement about Type 2 diabetes is true?

a. It develops rapidly.

b. There is a cure for the disease.

c. It occurs most often in those under 40.

d. Many people with the disease have no symptoms.

2. Tingling in the feet is one possible sign of which condition?

a. Retinopathy

b. Neuropathy

c. Nephropathy

d. Cerebrovascular disease

3. How can you lower your risk of getting Type 2 diabetes?

a. Lose excess weight

b. Get lots of sleep at night

c. Give up smoking

d. There is nothing you can do to lower your risk of Type 2 diabetes

4. Which statement about ``insulin resistance`` is most true?

a. It is caused by a virus.

b. It lowers the sugar levels in the blood.

c. The body can`t use the insulin that is produced.

d. It is a temporary condition.

5. Over the past 10 years, the prevalence of Type 2 diabetes has increased by what percentage?

a. 15%

b. 33%

c. 49%

d. 149%

6. You are caring for someone who has signs of mild hypoglycemia. Based on what you have learned, what should you advise this person to immediately consume?

a. 6 pieces of hard candy

b. 1 ½ cups of fruit juice

c. ½ cup of diet soda

d. ½ cup of skim milk

7. What advice would be most helpful for a person with Type 2 diabetes?

a. Avoid all unhealthy snacks

b. Walk around the house in bare feet

c. Avoid exercise until obesity has been controlled

d. See the doctor before beginning a new exercise program

ANSWERS

d. Many people with Type 2 diabetes have no symptoms.

b. Tingling in the feet is a possible sign of neuropathy.

a. Having extra weight, especially around the waist, is one of the risk factors for Type 2 diabetes. About 90% of patients who develop Type 2 diabetes are obese.

c. Insulin resistance is a condition in which the pancreas produces insulin but the body cannot use it.

c. The prevalence of Type 2 diabetes has increased by 49% over the past decade – a change that has been linked to the increase in overweight and obesity in the population.

a. Treatment for mild to moderate hypoglycemia consists of giving 15 grams of glucose (or carbohydrate that contains glucose) to an adult. 5-6 pieces of hard candy would be sufficient.

a. Encourage the person to stick to the meal plan and avoid all unhealthy snacks.

Tips for caring for the person
with Type 2 diabetes

1. Know the management plan.

2. Provide emotional support, especially when the person is first diagnosed.

3. Assist your family member to get education as needed.

4. Assist the person to test blood glucose levels as instructed.

5. Record blood test results, weight, and food eaten.

6. Encourage the person to control blood pressure, blood sugar levels, and cholesterol levels.

7. Encourage your loved one to stick to the meal plan. Help her find healthy foods.

8. Encourage your family member to participate in physical activities as planned. Help him find an enjoyable activity.

9. Encourage a positive mental attitude.

10. Encourage participation in stress-reducing activities.

11. Ensure good skin and foot care.

12. Inspect your loved one's feet and lower legs for cuts and signs of injuries.

13. Ensure footwear fits properly.

14. Know the symptoms of hypoglycemia.

15. Know the symptoms of hyperglycemia.

16. Ensure that a health professional is called if your family member shows signs of hypoglycemia or hyperglycemia.

17. Know the long-term complications that can develop with diabetes.

REFERENCES

American Diabetes Association. National diabetes fact sheet, 2005. Retrieved July 28, 2006, from http://www.diabetes.org/uedocuments/NationalDiabetesFactSheetRev.pdf

American Diabetes Association (ADA). Standards of medical care in diabetes. Diabetes Care, 28, S4–S36.

Anderson, D. (Ed.). (2002). Mosby's medical, nursing, & allied health dictionary (6th ed.). St. Louis, MO: Mosby.

Canadian Diabetes Association (2003). Clinical practice guidelines for the prevention and management of diabetes in Canada. Can J Diabetes, 27 (suppl 2).

Canadian Diabetes Association. Diabetes facts. Retrieved July 28, 2006, from: http://www.diabetes.ca/Section_About/thefacts.asp

Canadian Diabetes Association. Prediabetes: A chance to change the future. Retrieved July 28, 2006, from http://www.diabetes.ca/Section_About/borderline.asp

Canadian Diabetes Association. Type 2 diabetes. Things you should know. Retrieved July 28, 2006, from http://www.diabetes.ca/Section_About/type2.asp#type2

Ebersole P., Hess P., Touhy T. & Jett K. (2005). Gerontological nursing healthy aging. 2nd Ed. St. Louis: Elsevior Mosby.

Edelman, R. (2005). Obesity, Type 2 diabetes, and cardiovascular disease (CE Article). Nutrition Today, 40 (3), 119-123.

Moshang, J. (2005). Type 2 diabetes: Growing by leaps and bounds. Nursing Made Incredibly Easy, 3 (4), 20-34.

National Diabetes Information Clearinghouse. (2006). Am I at risk for Type 2 diabetes? (NIH Publication No. 06–4805). Retrieved August 14, 2006, from http://diabetes.niddk.nih.gov/dm/pubs/riskfortype2/index.htm

Stanziale Cohen, A. & Edelstein, E. (2005). Sick-day management for the home care client with diabetes. Home Healthcare Nurse, 23 (11), 717-724.

Vokey, S. & Peters, A. (2005). Diabetes mellitus, Type 2 – A review. eMedicine. Retrieved July 28, 2006, from http://www.emedicine.com/emerg/topic134.htm